MW01493852

EKG Interpretation

24 Hours or Less to EASILY PASS the ECG Portion
of the NCLEX!

Chase Hassen

Nurse Superhero

© 2015

Disclaimer:

Although the author and publisher have made every effort to ensure that the information in this book was correct at press time, the author and publisher do not assume and hereby disclaim any liability to any party for any loss, damage, or disruption caused by errors or omissions, whether such errors or omissions result from negligence, accident, or any other cause.

This book is not intended as a substitute for the medical advice of physicians. The reader should regularly consult a physician in matters relating to his/her health and particularly with respect to any symptoms that may require diagnosis or medical attention.

First, I want to give you this FREE gift...

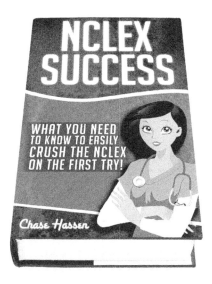

Just to say thanks for downloading my book, I wanted to give you another resource to help you absolutely crush the NCLEX Exam.

For a limited time you can download this book for FREE.

http://bit.ly/1VNGAZ9

Table of Contents

Introduction

I would like to thank and congratulate you for downloading EKG Interpretation. This book contains proven strategies and steps to understand the difficult details and components found in ECG tests which can give you a better understanding of the inner workings of the human heart.

Electrocardiography (ECG/EKG) has a core function of measuring the conduction system of the heart. It essentially involves a process of recording the electrical activities of the heart in a synchronized and right manner with the help of biomedical instruments.

When the cardiac muscles contract and relax, the myocardial cells which are present in the chest muscles get depolarized and repolarized. When the electrodes are placed on the body, these electrical changes get recorded on the graphing paper. This is called an ECG tracing and the dark horizontal line you see in the middle is the PQRST wave.

There are six chest leads ranging from V1 to V6, which helps in viewing the heart in the horizontal plane. Furthermore, there are electrodes affixed to the limbs that help in viewing the activities of the heart in the vertical plane. All 10 electrodes make up the 12-lead ECG placement and once synchronized together gives a good view on the condition of the heart.

In this book, we are going to discuss the details of the different parts of the PQRST wave and how an accurate and thorough analysis can help you understand the condition of the heart. With the knowledge we shall impart in this book, you will be in a better position in interpreting the rhythms of the heart. This is an excellent way of being aware of the state of the heart and ways by which you can handle the different aspects with clarity and understanding.

In order to provide proper patient care, you have to be mindful of how healthy the patient's heart is. Too often, even when we have the medical reports in front of us, we fail to understand what it means if we do not have the proper understanding and training for it. When you go through this book, you are going to gain a clearer understanding of what an ECG tracing denotes and be able to understand the core concepts of ECG as you work your way towards gaining a mastery of the heart.

Thanks again for downloading this book, I hope you enjoy it!

Chapter 1:
Electrical Conduction System

In order to familiarize with the concepts, we are going to talk about the key points that are in tune with the electrical conduction system. The heart muscles go through an electrical conduction system for the sake of generating an impulse. It is the sinoatrial (SA) node where the impulse kick-starts.

Once the impulse has been generated, it will then travel all the way through your cardiac muscles and thereby lead to muscular contractions.

The Sinoatrial (SA) Node

The SA node is responsible for generating the impulse in the heart. It is also known as the pacemaker and is found in the right atrium of the heart. The usual rate of this node varies from 60 to 100 beats per minute (bpm).

The Internodal Pathways

The heart is divided into two atria and two ventricles so there needs to be a connection between these chambers to ensure that the electrical impulse which is generated in the pacemaker can consequently travel through all the chambers. This is where the internodal pathways come in. The internodal pathways provide a passage which forms like a link between the SA node and AV node.

Located in the walls of the atria, these pathways aid in the conduction of impulses that run through the different parts of the heart.

The Atrioventricular (AV) Node

Located at the center of the heart, between the atria and the ventricles, this node has a huge role to play. It helps in slowing down the conduction rate of the impulse before it reaches the ventricles. This delay is extremely important for the sake of ensuring a smooth cardiac cycle. Due to this delay function, the atria can manage to eject blood completely before the ventricles start to contract.

Bundle of His

These are specialized heart muscle fibers, located in the inferior part of the interatrial septum, that aim to transmit the electrical impulses from the AV node to the left and right bundle branches in the heart.

Left Bundle Branch

As the name indicates, this branch helps in the conduction of impulse towards the left side of the heart muscles. These muscle fibers will lead impulses into the left ventricles and help in the initiation of the contraction there.

Right Bundle Branch

It serves the same use as the left bundle branch except it carries out the same action for the right side of the heart.

Purkinje System

The Purkinje System is located within the ventricular walls of the heart. These are extremely powerful fibers which can conduct the cardiac activity a lot quicker. These fibers are mainly known for their ability to cause synchronized contraction of the ventricles which ensures that the rhythm of the heart is consistent and well-maintained.

Depolarization and Repolarization

Depolarization is the process by which the electrical charge gets altered because of the changes in the electrolytes on either side of the cell membrane. Due to this charged effect, the muscles are forced to contract enabling depolarization to take place.

Repolarization on the other hand is the reverse process as the chemical pumps inside the cells reestablish the internal negative charge. This neutralizes the excess electrolytes making the muscles to return to their resting state.

Chapter 2:
Understanding ECG Tracing and How to Analyze the Rhythm

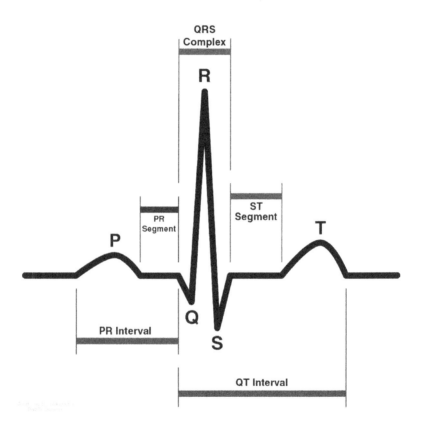

The ECG tracing is a combination of various waves, intervals, and segments that denote the condition of the heart. Here, you will get to see and understand what these different details and components represent and mean.

The P Wave

This is the first wave in the ECG tracing. It is a positive wave that is found in an upright position. The P wave denotes the depolarization and contraction of the atria. This wave represents the journey of electrical impulse generated by the SA node towards the moment when it reaches the right atrium and spans towards the left atrium via the Bachmann's bundle. This impulse is the one that causes the myocardium to contract.

The PR Interval

The PR interval is actually a representation of the delay which occurs in the AV node. This is an extremely important part of the ECG tracing. The lack of a PR interval could indicate that both the atria and the ventricles are contracting simultaneously. This simultaneous contraction hampers the smooth blood flow and can lead to heart-related complications.

This interval is a measure of the lag between the P wave and the QRS complex. It denotes or indicates the amount of time it takes for an impulse to travel from the atria to the ventricles.

The QRS Complex

The QRS complex actually has three clear deflections that follow after the P wave. They are an indication of ventricular depolarization and contraction. The Q wave is the first negative deflection on the tracing followed by the R wave which is a positive deflection and finally, the S wave with a negative deflection once more.

This part of the wave shows the journey of the impulse through the ventricular myocardium via the use of the right bundle fibers and the left bundle fibers. It also includes the rapid action of the Purkinje fibers which is responsible for the quick travel of electrical impulse throughout the heart muscles.

The ST Segment

The ST Segment measures the distance between the end of S wave and the start of the T wave. This segment measures the time gap between ventricular depolarization and the start of the repolarization phase.

The T wave

Just after the QRS complex you will find a small rounded upright wave. This is the T wave and it is an indication of the ventricular repolarization. Once the ventricles have been completely repolarized, they get ready for the start of a new cardiac cycle.

The QT Interval

This measures the time span from the start of the QRS wave to the end of the T wave. Thus, this interval will give you the complete duration of the ventricular activity during the cardiac cycle.

The U Wave

This is an extremely small wave which follows after the T wave. It is an indication of the repolarization of the Purkinje fibers and indicates that one cycle of the cardiac system is completed. This wave is more visible in tracings with a slower heart rate.

The Rate

The rate indicates the number of beats produced per minute, it is mainly a measure of the ventricular rate. In few cases, where the atria and ventricular rates differ, it is important to measure both rates. The normal rate lies within the range of 60 to 100 beats per minute.

In the case of bradycardia or slow heart rate, the number of beats per minute can fall down to less than 60 bpm while in the case of faster heart rates, it can go over the 100 bpm mark. Increased heart rate is a condition called tachycardia.

Regularity

Regularity is a component that measures the R-R intervals and the P-P intervals. If both of these intervals are consistent, it shows that the tracing is regular.

If there is a repeating pattern, it indicates that it is irregularly regular. However, if there is no specific pattern whatsoever, it means that the tracing is irregular.

Dropped beats

In some cases, the ECG tracings may show dropped beats. If this happens, it may indicate the presence of either a sinus arrest or an AV block.

QRS Complex Grouping

The QRS complex can be a good way to determine a lot of different abnormalities. This part of the tracing needs to be studied thoroughly to find what irregularities are present.

Here are some of the characteristics found in such irregularities:

If the QRS complex is normal but if it is followed by a premature complex, it indicates bigeminy.

If there is a repeating pattern of two normal complexes followed by a premature complex, it indicates trigeminy.

If there is a repeating pattern of three normal complexes followed by a premature complex, this is an indication of quadrigeminy.

If there are two consecutive premature complexes, this irregularity is referred to as couplets and there are three consecutive premature complexes this is called triplets.

Helpful Videos:

ECG 1 - ECG First Principles:

https://www.youtube.com/watch?v=tnJsol9sWfA

ECG 2 - P,Q,R,S & T Waves:
https://www.youtube.com/watch?v=3MRj8lheYDo

ECG 3 - Segments, Intervals & Diseases:
https://www.youtube.com/watch?v=XCmtP7597PI

Rate & Rhythm:
https://www.youtube.com/watch?v=F9yfo8-jRtY

Intervals & Segment:
https://www.youtube.com/watch?v=zFLg-J3XDpU

Chapter 3:
Sinoatrial (SA) Node Arrhythmias

The electrical conduction system of the heart is one of the many interesting aspects of the human body. It is a synchronized system of impulses and contractions that is responsible for supplying adequate blood supply for the human body. If one part falters in its function, it can drag down everything down with it over time.

The normal heart rate for a regular adult is 60 to 100 bpm and due to several intrinsic and extrinsic factors, it is prone to change depending on the applied stimulus and how the body reacts. On the case of arrhythmias, while some are quite manageable and not that serious, it is important to monitor the condition in case it takes a turn for the worse.

However, before we discuss the details of the different types of arrhythmias, let us take a moment to understand what an arrhythmia actually is. Arrhythmia, also known as dysrhythmia, is a type of condition where there is a problem on the formation and/or conduction of impulses within the heart thus leading to the alteration or disruption of rate and/or rhythm of the heart.

1. Normal Sinus Rhythm

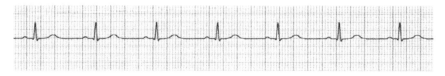

Now, before we talk about the different problems and complications, it is important to familiarize ourselves of what a normal heart with a regular rate and rhythm looks like. We call this condition, the normal sinus rhythm. This is where we can observe through the ECG tracing that the heart is functioning properly in terms of rate and rhythm.

This will be your basis as you take on the different complications and patterns found in ECG tracings. Also, please note that a normal ECG tracing will not necessarily rule of out a possible heart condition or disease.

How to detect the presence of a Normal Sinus Rhythm in an ECG tracing?

You will find that all the P waves look upright and similar. The PR intervals and QRS complexes have a normal duration of 0.12 to 0.20 seconds and 0.06 to 0.10 seconds respectively. The rhythm is even and there are no unwanted patterns or lags. If measured, the rate will range from 60 to 100 bpm.

2. Sinus Bradycardia

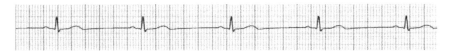

Bradycardia refers to slow heart rate. This occurs because the release of impulse from SA node is slower than normal which in turn causes the heart rate to slow less than 60 beats per minute.

Bradycardia essentially indicates that there is some kind of problem associated with the SA node. If the heart rate is terribly slow, the heart may not succeed in pumping blood to all the different body organs which can lead to very life-threatening complications.

However, it is important to note that a slow heart rate will not immediately signal a heart condition. Bradycardia is a common condition among athletes due to their increased vagal tone.

In fact, there are a lot of things that can cause sinus bradycardia like sleep, hypothermia, medication, increased intracranial pressure, and vagal stimulation like vomiting, suctioning, extreme emotions, and severe pain. It can also be caused by disease conditions like hypothyroidism and myocardial infarction (MI).

Also, while there people who do not really exhibit sign or symptoms of bradycardia, it is important to know that there are some (particularly those with pre-existing health conditions) that do experiences things like chest pain, fatigue, shortness of breath, weakness, syncope and confusion. Some may also complain of tiring easily during a physical form of activity.

How to detect the presence of Sinus Bradycardia in an ECG tracing?

If you look at the P waves, you will note that they are normal, uniform and upright. The PR interval is normal with duration of 0.12 to 0.20 seconds. The QRS complex is normal with duration ranging from 0.06 to 0.10 seconds.

Overall, the waves look normal, but if you calculate the rate, you will get a result of less than 60 bpm. If you compare the normal ECG tracing with that of bradycardia, you will find that in the case of bradycardia, the distance between the QRS complexes appear wider apart.

3. Sinus Tachycardia

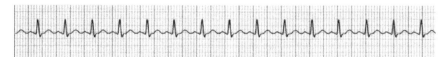

Tachycardia is a condition where the heart rate is higher than normal. Here, impulses speed up with the waves appearing more pronounced.

It is important to note that if the heart rate gets too fast, the overall efficiency of the cardiac cycle is going to decrease because the time taken by the ventricles to fill will be cut short.

There are various other factors which can also cause this medical condition. The heart rate tends to temporarily increase after extensive physical activities like exercise. It is also important to note that the heart rate tends to vary with age. Infants have an extremely high heart rate that gradually gets slower with maturation and age.

17

Possible conditions that can cause this are anemia, fever, anxiety, shock, hyper/hypovolemia, congestive heart failure (CHF), and hypermetabolic states. Patients who take sypathmomimetic medications are also prone to this condition.

While it is possible for people not to have any signs or symptoms when they have this condition, people experiencing sinus tachycardia may experience symptoms related to reduced cardiac output like low blood pressure and syncope. They may also experience dizziness, rapid pulse rate and shortness of breath. Some may even report feeling heart palpitations and chest pain.

How to detect the presence of Sinus Tachycardia in an ECG tracing?

If you take a close look at the tracing, you will find that the P waves are normal. There will be no abnormality with the QRS complex and the PR interval. The rhythm is regular, but the rate is going to be a lot faster.

You will also see that the waves are a lot closer to each other and the gap between the QRS complexes are significantly less, showing that the rate at which the cycle completes is reduced.

4. Sinus Arrhythmia

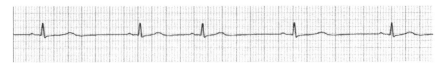

Sinus Arrhythmia as defined earlier pertains to a variation on the rate and/or rhythm of the heart. The rate of the heartbeat increases during inspiration and slows during expiration. While this condition does not make much hemodynamic effect and usually goes untreated, it can be caused (if no respiratory causes) by heart disease or a valvular disease.

How to detect the presence of Sinus Tachycardia in an ECG tracing?

In this medical condition, the distance between the two P waves increases. In this case, the SA node tends to discharge irregularly.

Even if you take a look at the R-R interval, you will find that it won't be regular either.

One of the best ways to diagnose the presence of this condition is to look at the P wave and check its presence. If it is present, but the waves are irregular, it indicates the onset of a sinus arrhythmia.

5. Sinus Pause (Sinus Arrest)

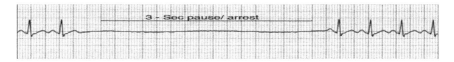

Sinus Pause is a medical condition wherein the SA node fails to generate an impulse for a certain brief period of time. Hence, you may observe a regular rhythmic pattern on the tracing and see a pause in between before the heart resumes once more.

There are many varying causes for sinus pause but they are usually attributed to diseases of the heart which in turn affects the functioning and health of the SA node. Medications like beta blockers and calcium-channel blockers can also cause this condition.

Most patients who suffer from sinus arrest often complain of dizziness and even palpitations. Sometimes patients can also collapse or pass out because of these irregularities and how it impacts the overall cardiac output. They may also complain of palpitations and flutters.

There are different treatments offered for this and the treatments are dependent on the main cause of the condition. One form of treatment is the insertion of an artificial pacemaker to ensure a steady heart rate.

How to detect the presence of a Sinus Pause in an ECG tracing?

This form of medical condition can be easily seen on the ECG tracings. If you look at the graph, you will find that there will be lack of waves signaling an arrest. The tracings will fail to show a regular pattern as there can be random moments of arrest that can delay or disrupt the heart cycle.

The electrical condition resumes either when the SA node is set into action again or if the latent pacemaker starts working as well. The pause or arrest time interval doesn't necessarily needs to be a multiple of the P-P interval and can have its own unique duration.

As we can see, the P waves are normal, but whenever an arrest occurs, they will disappear due to the occurrence of arrest. The rhythm becomes irregular as soon as the SA node fails to work. The rate is also going to fluctuate as well.

6. Sinoatrial (SA) Block

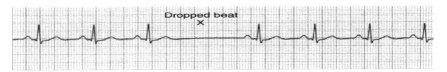

SA Block is a condition where the electrical impulse generated in the heart either gets delayed or blocked. This leads to the delayed depolarization of the atria. This is different from delayed ventricular depolarization because that is caused by an AV block. However, when atria fail to be depolarized, the reason lies in the irregular functioning of the SA node.

The causes for this condition are usually attributed to diseases that cause a deterioration and malfunction of the SA node like endocarditis, and coronary heart diseases. It can also be caused by medications like digoxin, beta blockers, and calcium-channel blockers.

Signs and symptoms of this condition usually depend on the severity of the SA block. Therefore, there will be some who are asymptomatic while others have symptoms associated with reduced cardiac output like syncope and dizziness.

How to detect the presence of a SA Block in an ECG tracing?

When you take a look at the ECG tracing, you will find that there will be dropped beats. The dropped beats will occur after a cycle.

After the dropped beat, the cycle resume once more. Furthermore, you can also see that the block actually occurs in multiples of P-P intervals. Expect a significant drop in cardiac output because of this condition.

You will notice that the P waves, PR intervals and the QRS complexes are normal except for the rhythm which can turn irregular due to the SA blocks. The rate can range from normal to slow.

There you go – the main categories sinus rhythms and their characteristics. These rhythms can be diagnosed and observed through careful and diligent study of ECG tracings. The more you are exposed to ECG readings, the easier it to find out whether the patient is suffering from these heart conditions.

Chapter 4:
Atrioventricular (AV) Blocks

Here, we will discuss the different types and degrees of AV blocks. An AV block is a medical condition which can be diagnosed by observing the ECG tracings properly. Those who are suffering from an AV block will find that there is impairment in the conduction of impulses from the atria to the ventricles.

Ideally, the SA node is responsible for setting the pace and regulating the speed of contraction. However, in the case of AV blocks, the ventricles fail to get the message from the SA node and while the ventricles come with their own pacing mechanism the heart rate gets slower because of this.

There are various causes of this condition and the common ones include drugs, infarction, ischemia and even fibrosis. AV blocks can be categorized under three different types which are the first, the second and the third-degree AV block.

First-Degree AV block

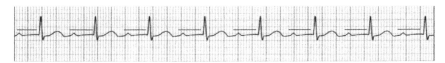

First Degree AV block is a medical condition where it is characterized by a noticeable PR interval prolongation for more than 0.20 seconds. In this medical condition, the impulse when traveling from the atria to the ventricle gets delayed because it travels slower than the normal speed.

The possible causes for this condition are enhanced vagal tone (especially in athletes and runners), diseases in the AV node, MI, myocarditis, medication or drugs, and electrolyte disturbances.

This degree of AV block is still generally asymptomatic and can only be detected through an ECG test. Usually, this condition is not that serious and is treated by most as benign. However, if accompanied with a case of acute MI, it can lead to some very serious AV defects, which can further aggravate the problem.

How to detect the presence of a First-Degree AV Block in an ECG tracing?

When you observe the ECG closely, you will find the following characteristics that shall denote the presence of this condition. There is no change in the P waves. The PR interval is longer as the duration is larger than 0.20 seconds. The QRS complex is normal and the duration would be between 0.06 to 0.10 seconds.

Second-Degree AV block

Similar to the first-degree AV block, this condition also denotes impairment in the conduction of the impulses from the atria to the ventricles. This condition occurs when more than one impulse fails to reach the ventricles.

The cause of second-degree AV block is usually attributed to the aliments and conditions that aggravate and damage the heart such as infections, metabolic disorders, heart disease, structural heart defects, and even medication.

Signs and symptoms for people vary since those experiencing Type 1 will more likely be asymptomatic than those who have Type 2. Those with Type 1 typically experience irregularities in heart rate while those with Type 2 experience syncope and bradycardia as well.

How to detect the presence of a Second-Degree AV Block in an ECG tracing?

Second-Degree AV block is split further into two subcategories namely type 1 (Mobitz I or Wenckebach) and type 2 (Mobitz II). While type 1 is a less serious case as compared to type 2, both of them has the condition on which the P wave is blocked from initiating the QRS complex.

Second degree type 1 block (Mobitz I or Wenckebach)

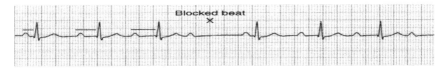

Here, you will find that the PR interval will keep on getting progressively longer, until you will see that a P wave gets totally blocked and no QRS was produced. There is a visible pause where the AV node recovers and the whole cycle starts over.

Second degree type 2 block (Mobitz II)

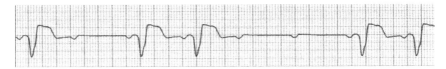

This type of block involves both the bundle branches. Here, if you take a look at the ECG, you will find that the distance between the P wave and the QRS complex gets wider with a conduction ratio that ranges from 2:1 to 3:1 or even 4:1. People with this type of heart condition are usually treated with artificial pacemakers to regulate their heart rates.

Third-Degree AV Block

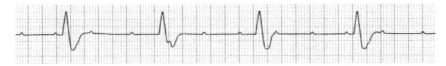

The third-degree AV block (also known as complete heart block) indicates a serious medical condition where there is something the causes a blockage of all impulses and prevents them from reaching the ventricles.

As the impulse gets blocked completely, the pacemakers in the ventricular chambers need to activate the ventricles so that the impulse can be generated. You would notice what this disharmony creates on the ECG tracings where the atria and the ventricles start to work independently to compensate for this electrical block.

While it is possible to have third-degree heart block due to a congenital defect, there are other possible causes that can lead to this condition like drugs, infection, rheumatic diseases, metabolic causes, and toxins.

Some who has this condition will be asymptomatic at first but the symptoms will eventually develop as the body fails to compensate. This condition usually has bradycardia, dizziness, chest pain, pulmonary edema, syncope, and confusion.

How to detect the presence of a Third-Degree AV Block in an ECG tracing?

The rhythms are regular, but both atria and ventricles will act independently. The P waves are likely to be normal but sometimes they get superimposed over the QRS complexes or the T waves. It is hard to tell anything about the PR interval as it tends to vary greatly.

Bundle Branch Block (BBB)

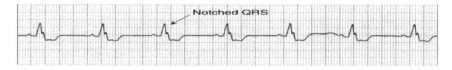

In this form of block, it is either the right or the left ventricle which gets late depolarization. Due to this late depolarization of either one of the ventricles, the QRS complex tends to get a notch.

Common causes for this condition are hypertension, infection of the heart muscle, congenital defects of the heart, pulmonary embolism and heart diseases. This condition can be asymptomatic and people may not even notice they have this condition. However, some do experience fainting or at least the feeling of about to faint.

How to detect the presence of BBB in an ECG tracing?

As observed in the tracing, the P waves and the PR interval are normal. The rhythm is regular as well. It is just that the QRS complexes which are wider and notched.

Helpful Videos:
> The ECG Course - AV Blocks:
> https://www.youtube.com/watch?v=nCZI_NY501Q

Chapter 5:
Atrial Arrhythmias

When arrhythmia occurs in the atria, we call them as atrial arrhythmias. Atrial arrhythmias come in different forms and complications. Therefore, it is best to familiarize yourself on how they differ from each other in terms of definition and appearance. Let us take a closer look at the details.

1.   Wandering Atrial Pacemaker (WAP)

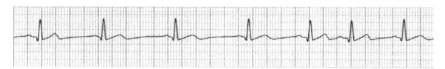

WAP is a condition that occurs when the natural pacemaker of the heart shifts to the different latent pacemaker sites. The pacemaker shifts away from the SA node and towards sites like the atria and the AV junction before shifting back to the SA node. This condition is almost never a cause for concern.

This condition is quite common in athletes, older adults, and young children. It can happen while exercising or sleeping. On rare cases, it can be caused by digitalis toxicity.

While there is a notable change in the ECG tracings due to the shifts, this condition does not require any kind of treatment and most patients do not even feel anything out of the ordinary when they have this condition.

How to detect the presence of WAP in an ECG tracing?

When you take a look at the tracings, you will find a noticeable change in the P wave which really differs from that of a sinus rhythm.

The P waves are likely to show at least three different forms which can be determined via the focus found in the atria. The PR interval varies and is determined by the focus as well. The QRS complex stays normal. While the rate will stay normal but will be paired by an irregularity in rhythm.

2.   Multifocal Atrial Tachycardia (MAT)

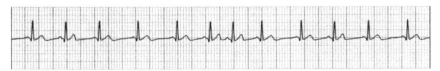

MAT is a condition that is mainly caused by a lot of electrical impulses sent from the atria to the ventricles. The condition can be associated with a ventricular response of more than 100 bpm and may be sometimes confused with an atrial fibrillation (A-fib) but unlike A-fib, MAT has a visible P wave, which can be observed in the ECG tracing.

Ideally, the rate of heart beat is controlled by the SA node which is the natural pacemaker of the heart. However, in the case of MAT, we will have different locations in the atria releasing impulses simultaneously. This simultaneous action triggers the heart to pump really fast resulting to an increase in heart rate which commonly ranges between 100 to 130 bpm causing inefeciency in the supply of blood flow.

The possible causes for MAT are coronary artery disease, heart failure, valvular heart disease, diabetes mellitus (DM), hypokalemia, hypomagnesemia, azotemia, sepsis, pulmonary embolism, pneumonia, and a postoperative state.

Patients with MAT experience signs and symptoms like fainting, chest pain, shortness of breath, palpitations, and lightheadedness.

How to detect the presence of MAT in an ECG tracing?

You will find at least three different waveforms of P waves which depend on the focus of the atria. The PR interval is going to vary and will depend upon the focus as well. The QRS complex stays normal but the rhythm turns irregular.

If you are wondering as to what would be the difference in graph for multifocal atrial tachycardia and wandering atrial pacemaker, the answer lies in the rate.

Look at both the graphs closely and you will find that in the case of MAT, the heart rate is quite rapid while in the case of WAP, the heart rate stays perfectly normal with the waves less closely spaced than the ones found in MAT.

3.   Premature Atrial Contraction (PAC)

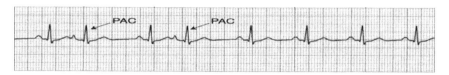

PAC is a medical condition that happens when the atria faces premature heartbeats. Premature heartbeats are seen as a complete ECG complex on the tracings which is due to the occurrence of an electrical impulse being released earlier than the next expected normal impulse of the SA node.

PACs are mostly caused by stress and intake of stimulants like coffee, tobacco, and alcohol. It may be caused by underlying cardiac conditions like hypertension, a previous MI, and a valve disorder. Also, electrolyte imbalances like abnormal blood levels of potassium and/or magnesium can cause it.

One symptom of PACs is usually sensations in the chest or a fluttering sensation. In most cases, this is not considered to be fatal and some may loosely refer to is as 'my heart skipped a beat'. However, if it occurs more frequently (more than six per minute), it may lead to further complications of a disease state or start a very serious arrhythmia like an A-fib and would require proper treatment and interventions.

How to detect the presence of PAC in an ECG tracing?

The P waves will be present, but when premature atrial contraction occurs, they are likely to develop a different shape. The PR interval stays normal; however, during the occurrence of PAC, you will find that the interval is going to vary significantly.

The QRS complex stays normal. If you look at the rhythm in the graph, you will find that the graph will show some irregularity, especially when a PAC occurs. The heart rate is also going to depend on the underlying rhythm and will likely vary.

4.   Atrial Tachycardia

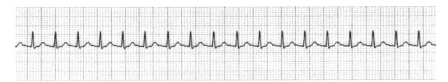

Atrial Tachycardia is a heart condition where the electrical impulse is generated somewhere in the atrial chambers as opposed to the SA node. In this condition, the SA node has been overridden and is no longer the dominant pacemaker. It is a type of supraventricular tachycardia (SVT) and does not needs the AV junction, the accessory pathways or even the ventricular tissue to function in terms of initiation and maintenance.

People with structurally abnormal hearts can have this problem but are less likely able to tolerate this type of rhythm abnormality unlike those people with normally structured hearts who have a lower mortality rate despite having this condition. Atrial tachycardia can occur with exercise, alcohol ingestion, hypoxia, metabolic disturbances, drug use, and acute illness.

Common signs and symptoms associated with the Atrial Tachycardia are sudden occurrence of palpitations, a rapid pulse rate, syncope, dizziness, dyspnea, pressure in chest, and even fatigue. Signs of heart failure may also be present as well as the occurrence of a warm-up phenomenon where the heart rate gradually speeds up soon after onset.

How to detect the presence of Atrial Tachycardia in an ECG tracing?

The P waves are normal, but they are different in term of shape unlike that of the sinus P waves. The PR interval tends to be short with a duration of less than 0.12 seconds during rapid rates. The QRS complex though normal tends to be irregular at times. Heart rate can be as high as 150 to 250 bpm with a regular rhythm.

On some cases, it can be observed that the ST wave and even the T wave can show signs of abnormalities as well.

5.   Supraventricular Tachycardia (SVT)

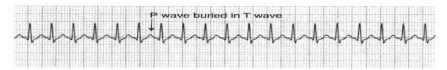

SVT is a case that involves an impaired electrical activity wherein the rhythm of the heart doesn't originate from the SA node; rather the action takes place above the heart ventricles and may even involve the AV node. There are two main types of supraventricular tachycardia which are as follows:

Atrioventricular nodal reentrant tachycardia (AVNRT)

Atrioventricular reciprocating tachycardia (AVRT)

Possible triggers or causes for this condition aside from heart ailments are medications, excessive drinking of caffeine and/or alcohol, smoking, and stress.

When you experience SVT, the heart tends to beat extremely fast and there are cases when the rate reaches as high as 150 to 250 bpm. However, it is important to note that people with have SVT may or may not experience obvious signs or symptoms. Some of the key symptoms of this medical condition are palpitation, pounding pulse, and/or dizziness. Other symptoms include syncope, shortness of breath, sweating, and chest pain.

Due to the increased heart rate, there is a possibility that people with this condition will likely develop heart failure. The risks are higher in those who have more frequent SVT episodes along patient that have a pre-existing heart condition.

How to detect the presence of SVT in an ECG tracing?

The P waves are going to be difficult to see and will often be buried inside the T waves. The PR interval cannot be measured. The QRS interval is likely to be normal but at times can be wide if abnormally conducted through the ventricles. The rhythm of the heart beat is going to be regular. You will find very closely spaced waves with a rate that can go as high as 150 to 250 bpm.

6.   Paroxysmal Supraventricular Tachycardia (PSVT)

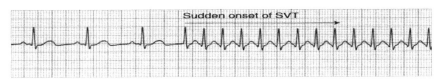

Stemming from the word 'paroxysmal' which means 'from time to time', PSVT is a condition that mainly occurs in the form of episodes characterized by a rapid heart rate that starts right about the ventricles. This type of condition starts and stops abruptly so in order to trace the presence of this abnormality, you must find and note the onset or end of the PSVT episode.

PSVT is generally not life-threatening but if there are other heart conditions present, it may lead to cases like Congestive Heart Failure (CHF) and/or angina. The form of treatment varies depending on the frequency of these episodes as well as if there is a presence of pre-existing diseases that may lead to further complications.

Possible causes for this condition can be hyperthyroidism, a previous MI, a mitral valve prolapsed, pneumonia, pericarditis, a chronic lung disease, and excessive consumption of stimulants like caffeine, drugs, and alcohol.

People who have this condition may experience heart palpitations, a feeling of tightness or pain in the chest, anxiety, and shortness of breath. A rapid pulse may also be felt upon assessment.

How to detect the presence of PSVT in an ECG tracing?

The P waves are going to be difficult to see and will often be buried inside the T waves. The PR interval cannot be measured, usually.

The QRS interval is likely to be normal but at times can be wide if abnormally conducted through the ventricles. The rhythm of the heart is going to be regular. The heart rate can rise to as high as 150 to 250 bpm.

As you must have noticed, the tracing is largely similar to SVT. However, one way to differentiate the two is through the presence of the rapid onset and termination of the episode.

7. Atrial Flutter (A-flutter)

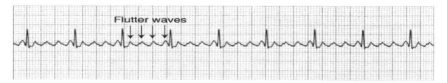

A-Flutter is a condition which mainly impacts the atria causing it to release impulses as much as 250 to 400 times per minute. This rapid atrial rate is too fast for the AV node, which means not all of these atrial impulses get conducted to the ventricle creating a therapeutic block at the AV node to prevent the heart from producing a ventricular rate as fast as 250 to 400 per minute leading to ventricular fibrillation, a very life-threatening arrhythmia.

One of the major troubles with this problem is the fact that owing to excessively high rate of heart beat, the heart may fail to pump ample blood and thus the different vital organs of the body will fail to get adequate blood supply.

People who have coronary heart disease may be at risk of developing this condition. This includes people who have undergone open-heart surgery, and/or have been exposed to a lot of stressors.

The patient with A-Flutter may complain of feeling faint, have shortness of breath, and pressure in the chest. A fast heart rate can also be observed.

How to detect the presence of A-Flutter in an ECG tracing?

The P waves have a distinct saw-toothed appearance. The PR interval is going to vary. The QRS complex is normal. However, if the flutter waves get buried in the complex, you may find them widened. The rhythm is regular and but that too can vary depending on the condition. When it comes to the heart rate, the heart rate is going to be pretty fast as it can vary from 250 to 350 bpm. The ventricular heart rate can be be slow or fast.

An important point to note is that an A-Flutter is mostly the first indication of any kind of cardiac trouble or ailment.

8.   Atrial Fibrillation (A-Fib)

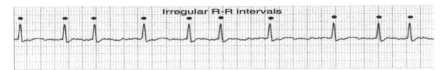

A-Fib is a condition wherein people experience irregular rapid uncoordinated twitching of the atrial cardiac muscles. This condition is one of the most common arrhythmias where people actually seek medical attention. It can occur in a paroxysmal basis or can become more chronic if left unmanaged. A-Fib, similar to PVST can start and stop in an abrupt manner.

There are many factors that can increase the risk of having an A-Fib – this includes hypertension, heart ailments, moderate to heavy alcohol intake and old age.

People who are experiencing A-Fib may complain of heart palpitations, chest pain, and shortness of breath. They may also feel lightheadedness, exercise intolerance, abdominal pain, and lack of energy.

How to detect the presence of A-Fib in an ECG tracing?

One of the most striking features has to be the absence of P waves. The whole segment of the tracing where the P waves are supposed to be present is extremely chaotic. There is no PR interval whatsoever. The QRS complex is normal and shows no signs of abnormality. The rhythm is irregular. The rate for the atrial segment is pretty high and can be as high as 350 bpm or even more. Ventricular rate can be either slow or high.

9.   Wolff-Parkinson White (WPW) Syndrome

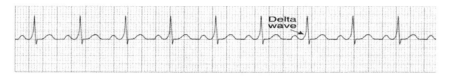

WPW is a syndrome which occurs because of the presence of an accessory conduction pathway between the atria and the ventricles. Due to this, pre-excitation occurs. Pre-excitation is an early activation of the ventricles because impulses have bypassed the AV node through the use of an accessory pathway. Such rapid impulses gives the initial portion of the QRS a notable slurring, this is called the delta wave.

There is little to know on the cause of WPW except that it is caused by a genetic mutation which is why it is common associated with those with congenital heart defects like Ebstein's anomaly.

Those with this case experience palpitations, dizziness, fainting, anxiety, and are easily fatigable. In severe cases, chest pains, difficulty of breathing, and sudden death (rarely) may happen. For infants, it can be noted with poor eating, lack of activity, shortness of breath, and fast heartbeats visible on the chest.

How to detect the presence of a WPW Syndrome in an ECG tracing?

If no A-fib is present, the P waves are going to be normal and upright. If the P wave is present, the PR interval will turn out short with a duration of less than 0.12 seconds. The delta wave is present, the QRS complex is going to be wide and may last for more than 0.10 seconds. The rhythm is regular, if there is no atrial fibrillation. The presence of an A-fib will turn the rhythm irregular. The rate will depend on the underlying rhythm

Helpful Videos:
The ECG Course - Atrial Rhythm:
https://www.youtube.com/watch?v=FtGiphQBuaI

Chapter 6:
Junctional Arrhythmias

Another type of arrhythmia is junctional arrhythmias which mainly focus on the problems found within the SA node and/or the atria which interfere with the normal pacemaker mechanisms of the heart.

On this chapter we will go tackle the different types of junctional arrhythmias and learn how to differentiate each irregularity from each other. This chapter would also include the common signs and symptoms being experience by client who have these types of heart rhythm irregularities.

1.   Junctional Rhythm (Idionodal Rhythm)

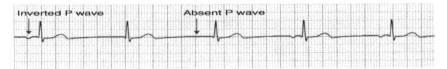

Junctional or idionodal rhythm is an abnormal condition of the heart which mainly arises when the AV node replaces the SA node at the pacemaker of the heart. This case can happen when something slows the SA node down or when an impulse fails to be conducted through the AV node, this failure would cause a junctional escape rhythm to begin as a compensatory response.

There are numerous causes for this condition to occur. It can be caused by acute inflammatory process that has compromised the conduction system of the heart like acute rheumatic fever. Further causes include drugs that can slow your heart rate as a side effect. Sick sinus syndrome, digoxin toxicity and diphtheria can cause junctional rhythms as well.

Now while some people with junctional arrhythmias are completely asymptomatic, some can experience palpitations, syncope, dizziness, dyspnea, and/or fatigue. So make sure to assess your patients properly.

How to detect the presence of a Junctional Rhythm in an ECG tracing?

If you try to look for the P waves, you would notice that they are either completely absent, buried, inverted or retrograde. The PR interval will be affected too. It can either be completely absent or become very short and retrograde as well.

In terms of the QRS complexes, they are going appear normal. The heart rate will be as slow as 40 to 60 bpm with a regular rhythm.

2.   Junctional Tachycardia

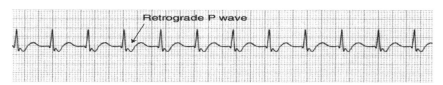

Junctional Tachycardia is type of SVT which involves the AV node. In this form of junctional disorder, the impulse is generated in focus in parts of the AV node instead in the SA node which causes abnormalities in heart rate.

This condition can be associated to digitalis toxicity and even indicate an onset of a heart ailment like acute coronary syndrome. Diseases like heart failure and ailments found within the conduction system leading to increased automaticity can cause this condition as well.

If you are looking for sign or symptoms, kindly remember that a decrease in cardiac output can occur due to the increased rate of the heart so watch out for those types of signs and symptoms.

How to detect the presence of Junctional Tachycardia in an ECG tracing?

While looking at the tracing, take note that the P waves like in the case of junctional rhythm are absent, inverted, buried, or are retrograde. The PR interval can be absent, short, or retrograde. The QRS complex is also normal. The only notable difference between a junctional rhythm and a junctional tachycardia is that the rate in junctional tachycardia would go as fast as 100 to 180 bpm.

3.   Junctional Escape Beat

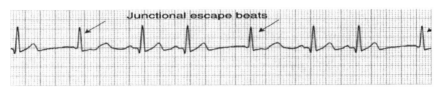

Junctional Escape Beat is a condition wherein the heartbeat originates not in the atrium but in an ectopic focus usually somewhere in the AV junction (like the Bundle of His). This mainly occurs when the rate of depolarization of the SA node falls below of what the AV node can offer.

This is mainly a protective mechanism used by the heart for the sake of compensating the inability of the SA node to handle the pacemaker activity. The possible causes for this condition the presence of sinus bradycardia or some high degree of AV block.

In terms of signs and symptoms, it is important to note that the client may experience symptoms of those that have bradycardia like syncope, dizziness and hypotension.

How to detect the presence of Junctional Escape Beat in an ECG tracing?

Similar to the previous junctional arrhythmias discussed, P waves in junctional escape beat are most likely completely absent, buried, inverted or retrograde as well. The PR interval can be absent, short, or retrograde. In addition, the QRS complex is not going to show any abnormalities. Take note that the rhythm will likely vary.

Also, it can be noted that the escape complex comes after or later than the next sinus complex.

4.   Premature Junctional Contraction (PJC)

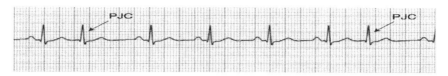

PJCs are premature cardiac impulses which originate near the AV nodal area or the AV junction of the heart. This occurs right before an impulse from the SA node can reach the AV node. This increased automaticity creates PJCs.

These types of beats can sometimes be seen even in healthy person are less common than PACs. The causes for PJCs usually involve a type of ailment or condition like digitalis toxicity, congestive heart failure, and coronary heart diseases. Other causes also include alcohol consumption, adrenergic stimulants and tobacco.

As stated earlier, there people despite being healthy, experience this. These people are usually asymptomatic. However, there are some cases the people palpitation and sometimes even experience synchronous contraction of the atria and ventricles. This occurrence is called cannon a waves. You can tell if a person might be experiencing this when you distressing pulsations on their neck.

How to detect the presence of PJCs in an ECG tracing?

Like most of the junctional arrhythmias, you will find that the P waves are going to be absent or even inverted, buried or even in the retrograde position. The PR interval is most likely absent, short or retrograde. The QRS complex of course, stays normal. The rhythm will show irregularity whenever a PJC occurs. The rate will depend directly upon the underlying rhythm of the heart.

As you have observed, junctional arrhythmias possess very similar characteristics in their ECG readings so make sure to carefully check and assess the other notable factors that make these ECG readings unique.

Helpful Videos:
Junctional Rhythms:

https://www.youtube.com/watch?v=wpE0-74eHbI

Chapter 7:
Ventricular Arrhythmias

What is a ventricular arrhythmia? As you now all know, arrhythmia refers to a disorder in the conduction and/or formation of electrical impulse in the heart which would lead to alterations in terms of rate, rhythm, or both. Therefore, when we talk of ventricular arrhythmias, it refers to a disorder which arises in the ventricular region of the heart.

Like on the previous chapters, we will cover the different types of ventricular arrhythmias and learn how to differentiate each irregularity from each other. Aside from that, we would also include the common signs and symptoms being experience by client who have these types of heart rhythm irregularities.

1.   Idioventricular Rhythm (Ventricular Escape Rhythm)

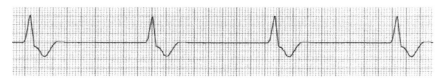

Idioventricular Rhythm happens when an impulse begins in a conduction system somewhere below the AV node. When the SA node was not able to generate an impulse, or when an impulse was generated but it was not conducted properly through the AV node, the Purkinje fibers compensate and automatically discharge an impulse. This condition can be also referred to as Agonal Rhythm.

Possible causes for a person to develop this type of heart rhythm is if they are have conditions like severe sinus bradycardia, a sinoatrial block, a high grade Second-degree AV block, and Third-degree AV block. Hyperkalemia, sinus arrest and medication like beta blockers and calcium channel blockers can also predispose to this condition.

Aside from bradycardia, signs and symptoms associated with decreased cardiac output like syncope can usually be seen in patients with idioventricular rhythm.

How to detect the presence of Idioventricular Rhythm in an ECG tracing?

The first thing to notice is that the tracing for this rhythm has no trace of P waves whatsoever. You would not see the PR interval either. The QRS complex comes with a bizarre look and you will find that there are extremely wide intervals between complexes as well. The duration could last for as long as 0.10 seconds. The rhythm is regular but the rate of heart beat can be as slow as 20 to even 40 bpm.

2.   Accelerated Idioventricular Rhythm (AIVR)

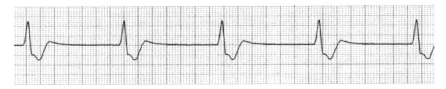

AIVR is a condition where the ventricular rate will stay between 41 to 100 bpm. This mainly occurs when the rate of generation of impulse by the ectopic ventricular pacemaker is going to exceed that of the SA node.

It is usually accompanied with an increase in the vagal tone and a simultaneous decrease in the sympathetic tone. This condition can be present in an athletic heart. However, there can be plenty of other reasons for experiencing this anomaly such as an acute MI (reperfusion phase), cardiomyopathics, CHD, myocarditis, medication (e.g. beta-sympathomimetics), electrolyte imbalances, drug toxicity (e.g. cocaine, digoxin, desflurane), and the return of spontaneous circulation post cardiac arrest.

Since this type of condition happens when supraventricular pacing sites get depressed or are absent, symptoms associated with reduced cardiac output are expected, especially if the heart rate is slow.

How to detect the presence of AIVR in an ECG tracing?

The ECG tracing is going to be extremely similar to that of idioventricular rhythm. This whole case is similar with the only difference of it being accompanied with an increase in heart rate.

The P waves are going to be completely absent as well as the PR interval. The QRS complex has an extremely strange appearance and when they occur, you will find them having a wide duration of greater than 0.10 seconds. The rhythm is regular but as stated earlier, the heart rate is going to be between 41 to 100 bpm.

3.   Premature Ventricular Contraction (PVC)

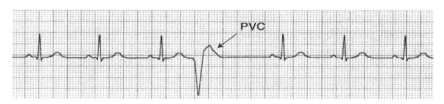

PVCs are termed so because they occur before a regular heartbeat. They are mainly caused when the beat occurs in a premature manner in the ventricles of the heart.

Here, the impulse is generated in the ventricle rather than the SA node and is conducted through the ventricles before the occurrence of a normal sinus impulse. Healthy people can experience PVCs and since some cases of premature ventricular contractions are benign, they will not require any kind of special treatment.

PVCs can be caused by caffeine, nicotine, and/or alcohol consumption as well as cardiac ischemia or infarction, digitalis toxicity, hypoxia and electrolyte disturbances like hypokalemia. It can also happen due to conditions that contribute to an increased workload of the heart like tachycardia, fever, exercise, heart failure, and hypervolemia.

It is important to note that PVCs in acute MI may indicate the need to for more aggressive forms of treatment. In addition, PVCs may also indicate the possibility of a ventricular tachycardia may occur.

PVCs are usually asymptomatic, especially for healthy individuals. However, there are cases when people who experience PVCs can feel odd sensations in the chest. They usually describe them as akin to skipped or missed beats, fluttering, pounding or jumping, flip-flops, or an increased awareness of your heart beating. These sensations are due to the fact that the ventricles are only partially filled. PVCs do not always generate pulses as well.

How to detect the presence of PVCs in an ECG tracing?

PVCs come in many forms, so it is important to take note of the presented ECG tracings and their descriptions. They can be classified into unifocal and multifocal. Unifocal means that each PVC is identical and came from a single ectopic focus. Multifocal comes from two or more ectopic foci thus making multiple QRS morphologies. Another term to classify PVCs is uniform (one form) and multiform (many forms).

You will also notice a pause following the PVC followed by a normal beat that arrives after an interval equal to twice the preceding R-R interval. This is called a full compensatory pause. However, note that these pauses can be noncompensatory as well.

However, despite the differences, PVCs still share some distinct qualities with each other. The QRS complex is wide with a span of more than 0.10 second and they will show a bizarre look. The rhythm of the heart will become irregular as soon as PVC occurs. The heart rate is also going to depend on the rate of the underlying rhythm.

Now, closely look at the two tracings to give you a nice overview on what a uniform PVC looks in comparison to that of multiform.

Uniform:

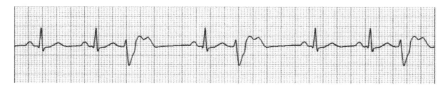

Multiform:

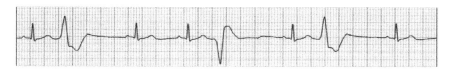

It is important to understand the difference between two forms. As the name implies, the multiform tracing shows different forms of beats and the graph has a lot more variation as compared to the former one which has the same pattern repeated all over it.

But wait, there's more. There are various other forms of PVC too. They are bigeminy, trigeminy, quadrigeminy and couplets.

As you can see in the tracings, ventricular bigeminy is the condition when people experience PVC for every other beat per cardiac cycle. Trigeminy will occur of PVC occurs after every third beat.

In a similar manner if people experience a PVC after every fourth beat, the situation will be termed as quadrigeminy. In some cases, the occurrence of paired PVCs can happen as well. Such a situation is called as couplets.

PVC: Ventricular Bigeminy:

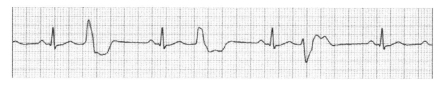

PVC: Ventricular Trigeminy:

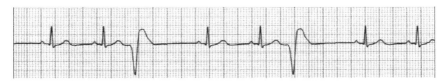

PVC: Ventricular Quadrigeminy:

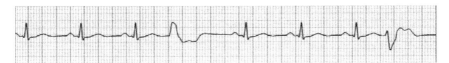

PVC: Couplets:

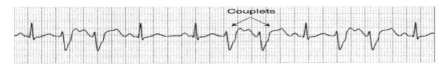

Ventricular tachycardia (VT)

VT is a kind of medical problem where three or more PVCs in a row happen with the heart rate exceeding 100 bpm. The rhythm may arise from the ventricular myocardium, the distal conduction system of the heart or even both.

The possible causes for VT are cardiomyopathies, heart surgery, myocarditis, a valvular heart disease, and heart failure. This condition may even signify an early or late complication of a heart attack. People without heart problems or ailments can have this condition as well.

VT episodes are quite fast and may last longer than a few seconds. Patient having an episode may experience angina, shortness of breath, palpitations, dizziness, and syncope. Symptoms for VT may start and stop in an abrupt manner. Sometime, there may not be even symptoms to serve as a warning.

How to detect the presence of VT in an ECG tracing?

Based upon the morphology, VT can be of two different types namely, monomorphic and polymorphic.

Monomorphic Ventricular Tachycardia

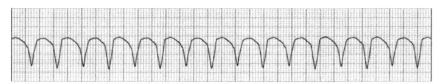

As the name implies, monomorphic means that the different beats which you will spot on your ECG are going to match each other as they all carry the same form.

The P wave is not going to be present at all. There is no PR interval either. The QRS complex is bizarre in shape and has a span more than 0.10 second giving it a wide appearance. The rhythm though regular, you will find the rate to be between the range of 100 to 250 bpm.

You should always make it a point to detect the presence or absence of pulses in response to the detection of this ECG tracing because monomorphic VT can be perfusing or even nonperfusing as well. If left untreated, monomorphic VT can eventually lead to ventricular fibrillation.

Polymorphic Ventricular Tachycardia

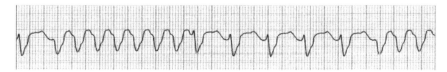

In this form of tachycardia, there are going to be various variations per beat. There is no uniform beats in the graph. If you look at the tracing, you can see that there are various progressive changes per cycle. The QT interval in this abnormality is either normal or long. The P waves are going to be absent or they won't be associated with the QRS complex. There will be no PR interval whatsoever. Like other waveforms, the QRS complex is going to have a strange look and the duration will be wide spanning for more than 0.10 seconds.

The rhythm can be both regular and irregular and the rate of heart beat is going be higher as it will be in the range of 100 to 250 bpm. When you look at both the monomorphic and polymorphic ECG tracings side by side, you will understand how the beats are going to vary for the two conditions.

1.   Ventricular Fibrillation (VF)

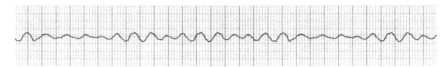

VF is mainly a condition where the cardiac muscles located in the ventricles of the human heart contract in a rapid and uncoordinated manner. The ventricles fail to contract properly. They merely quiver which means that the efficiency of the heart to pump blood is going to be impacted.

The causes for VF are similar to that of VT. In fact, untreated or unsuccessfully managed VT can lead to VF. Other possible causes for VF include electrical shock and the Brugada syndrome.

The Brugada syndrome is in which a person, usually of Asian descent, has a normally structured heart, few or no risk factors for Coronary Artery Disease, and a family history of sudden cardiac death.

Symptoms for VF include dizziness, shortness of breath, a rapid fluttering heartbeat, nausea, and chest pain. Eventually, the pulse would disappear along with the cardiac output. VF is an emergency situation and requires immediate attention because if left untreated, it will lead to death.

How to detect the presence of PVCs in an ECG tracing?

The electrical impulse which travels is very chaotic and there is no ventricular depolarization or contraction at all. You can find no trace of P wave, the PR interval or even the QRS complex. It is impossible to determine the rate of the heart beat and the rhythm is indeterminate. The only things distinguishable are the amplitude and frequency of the fibrillatory activity which can be defined as coarse, medium, or fine.

2.   Pulseless Electrical Activity (PEA)

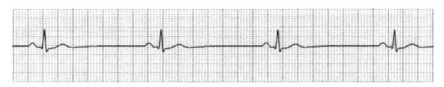

PEA, also known as electromechanical dissociation (EMD), is a condition where the heart fails to produce a pulse. In this medical condition, there is an electrical activation and the impulse is generated, but the heart muscles fail to contract.

The possible causes for PEA are pulmonary embolism, tension pneumothorax, electrolyte imbalances (e.g. hyper/hypokalemia), MI, hypovolemia, acidosis, hypoxia, hypothermia and overdose of drugs like beta blockers, digoxin and cyclic anti-depressants.

Signs and symptoms found in the case of PEA include the lack of heart tones upon auscultation, apnea and the lack of a pulse.

How to detect the presence of PEA in an ECG tracing?

If you take a look at the ECG tracing you would note that despite the presence of an electrical activity, everything from the rate, rhythm, P waves to the PR interval and QRS complex reflect only the underlying rhythm.

3.   Asystole

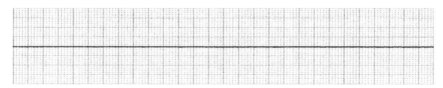

Also termed as 'flat line', asystole is a condition where there is absolutely no cardiac activity. This is a state where there is zero cardiac activity and no impulse is generated. Neither atria nor the ventricles are contracting and thus there is zero blood flow.

Asystole can be categorized by primary and secondary. Primary happens when the heart's conduction system intrinsically fails to generate ventricular depolarization resulting to the degeneration or ischemia of the SA or AV conduction system. Possible causes for primary asystole includes the proximal occlusion of the right coronary artery and extensive infarction.

Secondary asystole happens when extrinsic factors cause a malfunction on the heart's electrical conduction system causing a failure in the generation of any electrical depolarization. Possible causes for this includes near-drowning, stroke, suffocation, and MI complications.

A CPR must be performed at the earliest in order to rescue the person or else it can lead to instant death because the blood supply to vital parts of the body will be cut off. Sometimes, electric shock needs to be administered as well to get the heart working again. It is important to trace the main cause that has led to asystole as it is going to help in a speedy treatment. It is advised to check the ECG by performing it under two different leads to confirm.

How to detect the presence of asystole in an ECG tracing?

The ECG is going to show one flat line with no electrical activity whatsoever.

Helpful Videos:
>Ventricular Rhythms:
>https://www.youtube.com/watch?v=L83yVPXilSk

Conclusion

We are now at the end of your ECG learning journey. We have tackled and discussed the various types of heart rhythms and how they would appear in an ECG tracing. We have discussed their possible causes as well as the signs and symptoms that accompany them. We have offered you an exhaustive coverage of almost all possible types of arrhythmias which we hope means that you now have a good steady understanding on the subject.

We are confident that this book has helped you gain a great deal of understanding on the different ECG waves and intervals and how together, allows you an overview on how the heart is operating and its condition.

It is important to have a clear idea about the different waves, patterns, rhythms and rates as observed in the graph because this will improve your understanding of your own heart. Those who can read and understand the ECG are much more likely to be well acquainted with their patient's heart condition.

Make sure to use this book in the best manner. Grasping all the information at one go might be a little daunting and this is why you can go through it in parts and series as it will help you pick the right details. There are so many things an ECG reading can show you. Take your own time to surf through the pictures and correlate it with the information we have offered. We are sure this book will be the ultimate guide which will help you master and understand the wonders of the ECG!

Feel free to go through this book as many times as needed. Remember, practice makes perfect.

If you enjoyed this book, would you be kind enough to leave a review on Amazon? Your positive reviewers can help others to see what kinds of helpful resources are out there!

If you would like to be updated when each one of my new books come out, I will send you an email when it goes on free promotion! Just visit this link: http://bit.ly/1jqOAmG

I'll talk to you soon and see you in the next book!

Thank you and good luck on your medical endeavors!

- Chase Hassen

Nurse Superhero

Made in United States
Orlando, FL
28 April 2025